I0442029

How to Lose Weight: The Healthy Way

Jake Allen.

1

© 2015 Jake Allen.

All rights reserved. No part of this book may be reproduced or copied, except for review purposes.

Table of Contents

Introduction

It's a familiar story. You're reading a magazine or watching TV and you see a well-toned, fit model on the screen. You begin wanting to 'get in shape', just like these people you see all over the media. You visualize yourself being them, and you start planning your workout regimen and trying to eat less. But after a few days in, you revert back to your old ways, sitting on the couch, watching TV, and eating junk food, jealously looking at skinny people on TV and thinking negatively about yourself.

Okay maybe that's not exactly your story, but it's a common one told over and over. And it was my story.

I used to be overweight. My BMI was 27 so I kept trying to diet to reduce my weight to a healthy level. But what would always happen was that after skipping out on a few meals, I'd fail and overeat instead, and I'd always go back to indulging in my cravings. It was a terrible cycle as it kept making me feel inadequate, unable to stick with plans, and unable to fix my health situation.

But instead of giving up, I started studying more about how to lose weight in a more healthy manner. Rather than skip out on meals, I'd replace certain foods with healthier alternatives. I created a food log of the meals I was eating, and I started waking up early and exercising consistently. I'd set goals and plans that I'd make sure to follow through with, and I'd visualize the healthier me to stay motivated, until that version of me was realized. These steps helped me get to a normal BMI, to a state in which I was happy with myself and my body. I felt healthier and more lively.

From my experience, I wanted to outline the things I've learned and give you a quick guide to taking a healthier approach to food, exercise, and life. I'm here to teach you how to love yourself by eating right and exercising regularly. I want to teach you how to lose weight the right way. This requires, first to examine your lifestyle and identify how you can change it for the better.

So let's get into how to start losing weight the proper way!

Obesity and its Major Causes

According to the American Council on Exercise, to lose one pound of fat, you need to burn a whopping 3,500 calories. Weight loss ultimately comes down to one simple equation: if you eat more calories than you burn, you'll gain weight. If you eat fewer calories than you burn, you'll lose weight. It sounds easy, but it's obviously a lot harder than you'd think. A lot of people have problems trying to lose weight in a healthy way as well, for example they try to stop eating, or eat certain foods that don't have the right nutrients for the body. Weight loss is difficult, especially when it comes to making it a lifestyle that you can sustain.

So how do you know if you're in the danger zone when it comes to a healthy body mass index? To understand this, it's important to know what it exactly means to be obese or overweight. It's crucial to understand that being obese and being overweight mean two different things. Obesity means having excessive body fat that could result in a negative health impact, whereas being overweight means weighing more than what's considered normal, which doesn't have to mean excess fat. An obese person has a BMI (body mass index) of over 30 while an overweight person has a BMI of 25 and 29.9. A normal BMI is around 22.

Here, we'll list out some major causes of obesity.

Genetics
According to research, genetics plays an important role in chance of obesity. Part of the cause of obesity can highly depend on the medical history of the individual's family. The risk is two to eight times higher for a person with a family history in obesity as opposed to a person with no family history in obesity.

Lack of Physical Activity

Obesity is normally caused by eating too much and moving too little. Considering real life situations, 70% of jobs involve a minimum of 8 hours/day sitting. That's a LOT of time spent not moving. A study was shown that runners who take part in these job roles actually have side effects from sitting so much. Sedentary activity creates a lot of health problems. Rather than sit the whole day, try to stand up and walk around as much as possible. Try to get at least 1 hour of exercise in per day.

High Intake of Calories

It requires self control and determination to stop consuming too many calories. Try to only eat when you're hungry. However, don't NOT eat in an unhealthy way. 80% of us tend to leave our stomachs empty for more than 2 hours. Instead of doing this, always try to feed yourself small portions of healthy food every 2 hours a day. This will actually help prevent yourself from having cravings for junk foods like your favorite chips and candy.

Have you ever wondered how many calories you're consuming on a daily basis by drinking your favorite beverages? Sweet, sugary drinks are very high in calorie intake, including orange juice (110 cal), a medium mocha (400 cal), Coca Cola (280 cal), and sweet tea (200 cal). Consuming alcohol is another unhealthy habit that is costly in terms of calorie intake, e.g. beer is around 150 calories. It seems like everything that tastes good is bad for you, right? We'll get into how to combat cravings and identify healthy food substitutions.

Lack of Sound Sleep

Having a good amount of sleep serves you in numerous ways. It is recommended by experts to have a minimum of seven to eight hours of sleep a day for a healthier lifestyle, with 8 hours a day being optimal sleep.

Now, you should understand what causes unhealthy weight gain. To change these habits it's essential to write down your goals so you will have clear objectives and an action plan to get there, which we will talk about in the next section.

Goal Setting

Before jumping into your weight loss journey, you'll need to write down clear objectives regarding your fitness goals and what you are planning to achieve. You should be crystal clear about what you want - whether it be losing weight, building muscle, increasing stamina or anything else.

S.M.A.R.T. Goals

To create good goals is to create S.M.A.R.T. goals. S.M.A.R.T. goals are specific, measurable, attainable, realistic, and timely. Specificity and measurability are very important, reason being that you can easily know if you've accomplished your goals or not with specific detailed objectives that have time deadlines. Setting big fitness goals and accomplishing them are two different stories. If you set something unrealistic like a goal to lose 60 pounds in 1 month, it will ultimately lead you nowhere. Same is the case with dieting. You can't just tell yourself "I'm only going to eat 1 meal a day" and expect it to pan out long term. These goals are unrealistic and therefore not going to last. Make sure the fitness goals you are attempting to achieve are within limits and followed through in a healthy manner.

Some good examples of S.M.A.R.T. goals would be "I will lose 15 pounds in the next 3 months" or "I will reduce my body fat by 10 percent within the next 3 months". These goals are specific, measurable, achievable, and time-bound. They're also relevant to what you care about. Goals should always be important to you - not to your peers. Make sure your goals drive an intrinsic rather than extrinsic motivation to improve yourself.

Break Goals into Smaller Milestones

If you're using the goal of "I will lose 15 pounds in 3 months", you should create smaller S.M.A.R.T. milestones underneath these overarching goals. These milestones will help you achieve your bigger picture goal. For example, you can set S.M.A.R.T. goals for your eating habits. This could include "I will drink water instead of soda every week for the next 2 months" or "I will bring lunch instead of eat out for 4 days a week for the next 3 months". Set these goals for your fitness exercises as well, for example, "I will start doing cardio for 30 minutes a day, 3 days a week. I will commit to this for the next 2 months."

Develop a Habit of Writing Down Goals
One way of making yourself accountable for your goals is to write them down. Write down any of the goals you want to achieve, whether they revolve around fitness or around your other life domains. The act of writing something down subconsciously makes you more dedicated towards that goal just cause you've solidified it and made it more tangible. The thing about writing down your goals is that to do it, you have to have thought through and organized your ideas to formulate them onto paper.

Furthermore, writing down your goals somewhere you'll see regularly will act as a reminder on a daily basis. It's very easy to forget your goals if you've just formulated them in your mind. Try pinning a piece of paper with your written objectives in an area you will most frequently visit, like your closet, fridge, or bathroom mirror.

Go grab a pen and piece of paper right now! Write down your S.M.A.R.T. goals. What will you achieve, and when will you achieve them? Write down the overarching goals and the smaller milestones to reach those goals. Then stick the piece of paper on your fridge and make sure to follow it. It takes at least 3 months to really feel and see the difference, so don't lose hope and determination. All you need to do is stick with your goals step by step and try not to push for too much too soon!

Examples of Weight Loss S.M.A.R.T. Goals
In terms of overall S.M.A.R.T. goals you can set, here are some reasonable examples you can try out:

Weight: Aim for a weight loss goal of 1-2 pounds a week for at least a month. Even if you lose more the first week, don't expect it to last. The milestones should be gradual rather than all at once, as you want to keep with your lifestyle change instead of falling into a relapse.

Body Fat: A reasonable body fat loss goal is reducing by 0.5% a week. A sample goal would be: "I will lose 6% of body fat by 12 weeks."

Food Diary: Start documenting the amount of calories you're intaking and the foods you're eating. Hopefully after putting down a SMART goal you'll be more keen to keeping the habit permanently. A sample goal would be: "I will document every meal on the food diary every day for 1 month."

Leave Behind the Diet Mentality

If we're going to try and meet our S.M.A.R.T. goals, we have to start thinking right and eating right. Many people have this skewed notion that they need to restrict themselves from eating, but I recommend that you leave behind the diet mentality. So what IS the diet mentality?

The diet mentality involves this predictable thought process and cycle: we think that we should go on a diet and eat less so we can consume less calories. Following the equation that consuming fewer calories than you burn equals losing weight, it makes sense to want to diet and eat less.

But here are the problems with this idea:

Eating Less Pushes You to Eat More

You tell yourself you can never touch your favorite foods. Obvious, right? But with this plan, you normally won't be able to get all the nutrients needed for your body. You're also not getting enough calories to fuel your body which will push your body into a state of panic. The body's need to have sufficient fuel and nutrients is so powerful that you'll start developing cravings.   When you start thinking of junk food and sugary foods as "forbidden", it will amplify these cravings even moreso. Your brain starts thinking these foods are in short supply, making them even more appealing.

A lot of times what ACTUALLY happens when people try to maintain a diet mentality is that they quit the diet and start heading towards the opposite extreme, AKA they start indulging themselves in their forbidden cravings to the max. When your cravings are strong enough, it can make you jump to the other side of the fence. A lot of people will say "I quit the diet, so I might as well eat everything I wasn't initially allowed to."

Psychological Results of the Diet Mentality

By going on diets then failing to stay consistent, many people will start experiencing feelings of guilt and self-loathing. It's too common that people will feel bad about not continuing their diet, try to commit again, and predictably fail yet again. Diets will not only backfire but impact your emotional and mental state negatively.

The Solution?

Don't be one of those caught in this negative cycle! This restrictive and undesirable mentality sets us up for failure. That's the problem - we're setting ourselves up to switch back and forth from malnourishment and deprivation to excessive eating.

Start accepting the fact that diets rarely work. Diets are normally followed for a month or less and switched back to overeating again. Opt for a more tactical and realistic approach towards weight loss. Instead of participating in this cycle, start participating in supportive eating. Supportive eating involves regularly balanced meals that stops hunger while providing adequate nutrition that allows for a healthy lifestyle.

It's important to switch your weight loss mentality to a healthy one, but it will still require a lot of discipline, hard work, and consistency. Don't think there's an easy solution - you'll still need to dedicate yourself to exercise, follow through with goals, and replace excessive amounts of junk foods with healthier foods. In the following section, we'll start diving into what makes for a healthy eating lifestyle. We'll also talk about how to suppress cravings and control your diet by replacing foods and following specific tips.

Tips & Tricks to Help You Eat Healthy and Block Cravings

In this section, I want to provide some of the healthy eating tips and routines I use day to day. I'm also going to cover some healthy foods that you can use to replace your cravings. It might take a while to make new habits a part of your daily routine. But once you've introduced and developed practices to your lifestyle, you will see its positive effects very clearly.

Maintain a Personal Food Diary

As previously said, keeping a diary to log your day-to-day meal consumption helps remind you to go for healthier food options and think twice when following your cravings. To maintain this diary, you should create columns for every day of the week and rows for meals (breakfast, lunch, dinner). Start logging what you eat and drink every day. The food diary helps with weight loss through 2 means: awareness of what you eat and identification of possible patterns of overeating.

People who keep food diaries end up eating approximately 15 percent less food than those who don't. A researcher showed that people who keep a food diary 6 days a week lost about twice as much as those who kept food records 1 day a week or less. Put down a S.M.A.R.T. goal of practicing this every week for 3 months and see if there are significant results. If there are, don't stop there - keep doing it consistently to reach your goals.

Eat in the Early Morning

This is another tip that sounds counter-intuitive at first. Eating breakfast in the morning sounds like it would just add calories, so why eat that meal? The reason why eating breakfast is good is that it helps keep your metabolism high. Try to eat within 30-60 minutes of waking so that you can maintain a high metabolism and not feel starved later in the day (as this may lead you to bad decisions for lunch or dinner). If you're not a breakfast person, you can try drinking a smoothie or eating a piece of bread instead.

Along the same lines, it might actually be good to eat a donut with a high protein breakfast. Research on this was done with two test groups. One group ate a high protein 600 calorie breakfast along with a sweet, high carb treat (like a cookie, donut, or chocolate). The other group consumed a high protein 300 calorie breakfast. Surprisingly, the first group that consumed more calories wound up losing more than 37 pounds than the second group over a span of 32 weeks. Researchers found the reason behind this was that the desserts helped reduce hunger and cravings throughout the day.

Eating in the early morning with occasional sweets has helped me a lot in losing weight. By eating breakfast, I'm less tired and less hungry throughout the day.

Turn Away from Mouth-Watering Commercials
Try to switch channels when commercials of your favorite foods come in between your shows (or turn off your TV). Sometimes merely seeing food, even when on screen, can tempt and hinder you from achieving your weight loss goals. Studies have revealed that seeing high calorie foods stimulates the brain's satiety center, thereby spiking your hunger.

Hide Your Favorite Guilty Pleasure Foods
Hiding your favorite foods sounds almost too simple to be effective. However, a study showed that women who kept cookies or chips handy on their kitchen counters weighed around 10 pounds more than women who didn't.

My first tip would be to not buy too many junk foods when visiting the grocery store. Create a S.M.A.R.T. goal, for example, of not buying more than X amounts of cookies for every grocery run you make in the next 2 months. The reason behind this is that when you're hungry at home and you don't have any guilty pleasure foods within reach, you'll be less likely to take the trip to the store to get more cause it's so far away.

You should try your best to keep your food away from grabbing distance, so that you have time to think before reaching for them. If your chips and

What You Should Eat

We've gone over how to put goals in place and what different techniques you can use to stop yourself from eating when you aren't hungry. Now I want to cover the foods you SHOULD eat. Research shows that natural, unprocessed foods that humans are adapted to eat are good for health. For a balanced diet, your daily consumption should include some of the following healthy eating options:

Meat: Meat that has never been pumped with drugs and was given natural foods to eat is healthy. Consume white chicken or turkey meat as it is lower in fat than dark meat, red meat, and pork. Try eating ground sirloin or pork tenderloin. Unprocessed meat is good - meaning no bacon or sausages.

Fish: Fish is very healthy and should be eaten every week, preferably fatty fish like salmon. It is rich in omega 3-fatty acids and other nutrients.

Eggs: I personally don't like eating eggs (I'm weird like that) but they are very nutritious.

Vegetables: Eat vegetables every day. Vegetables contain fiber and other essential nutrients for the body.

Fruit: Load your bowl with healthy fruits like apples, bananas, pears, pomegranates, and oranges. Fruits are great because they taste good and are easy to prepare, and they're rich in fiber and Vitamin C. Eat in moderation though as they are high in sugar.

Drink Warm Honey Lemon Water

Boost your mornings with a mug full of hot water topped with honey and lemon. This is a good tip that will help energize you naturally, cleanse your entire bodily systems, nourish the body with vitamins, as well as quench your thirst and suppress hunger like none other. By incorporating this daily into your morning diets, you'll see dramatic benefits that aren't limited to weight loss.

Drink Matcha Tea

Matcha tea is green tea which helps boost metabolism and contributes in burning excessive fat from your body. The high levels of antioxidants in matcha are proven to be cancer-preventing and immunity-boosting. In one study, this tea was shown to lower risk of developing type 2 diabetes by 33 percent because it reduced blood glucose sugar levels. Unlike other drinks including coffee and other weight loss products, it won't over-stimulate the adrenal glands.

Start replacing your daily coffee or ginger tea fix with matcha tea. For a change of taste you can try mixing some lemon into it. It's stated that one glass of matcha tea is the equivalent of 10 green teas in its nutrients. So at the same time, make sure not to drink more than two cups on a daily basis, as over-consumption is never good.

Add Spice to Your Regular Meals

Adding some spices to your regular meals may contribute to weight loss. Research shows that Capsaicin (a chemical present in chilli peppers) activates your sympathetic nervous system which in turn speeds up your metabolism for more than four hours.

Brighten Up Your Meals

Try to load your plates with brightly colored fruits and vegetables as they are rich in nutrients essential for your body. By eating fruits and vegetables of different colors, you'll get the best all-around benefits as each color contains specific nutrients important to health. Various recent studies showed that people who have diets full of red, orange, and yellow vegetables and fruits had on average, smaller waists in comparison to those who didn't include these in their diet. To try this, you can for example top your fish entrees with a mango salsa or even sprinkle diced red pepper on top of your turkey meatballs.

Soup for Dinner

Celebrity trainer Joel Harper recommends serving up soups for dinner. In terms of digestion, he mentions that "liquids are already broken down," which means you have reduced the overall work which your body is supposed to do when breaking down foods. This will help make your weight-loss goals more attainable. With this method you'll need to focus on the quality of your calories and the health nutritional facts of your soup dinners. Some good soups to make include ginger-carrot soup, which is extremely rich in vitamin A, vitamin C and manganese, which helps in digestion. White bean pesto soup is also great and is composed of potatoes, beans and carrots. The soup demands approximately an hour of cooking time, but offers nine grams of fiber and less than 230 calories per serving.

What You Shouldn't Eat

By now you should be informed of what foods you should eat and tips to follow to help you in your goals. Now, we want to cover what you SHOULDN'T eat. By avoiding these drinks and foods you can make a dramatic difference in your healthy weight loss experience. Your body will thank you as consuming less of these foods means less chance of diseases and harm to your body.

Here are some of the following foods to avoid:

Sugar: Added sugar is addictive, so cut down on chocolates, candies, and other sugary treats. Foods with added sugar can be highly fattening and can cause diseases like obesity, cardiovascular disease, and obesity.

Grains: If you want to lose weight, you should try eating less bread and pasta. Gluten grains like wheat, barley, and rye are not good to consume for losing weight, but healthier grains like rice and oats are better to eat. You need carbs for energy so completely ridding yourself of grains from your diet is not the solution. It's about choosing the right carbs to get the balanced diet you need.

Artificial Sweeteners: These sweeteners are heavily correlated with obesity and other diseases.

Trans Fats: Chemically modified fats are extremely bad for health and found in processed foods, like fast food burgers and fries.

Highly Processed Foods: Highly processed foods like bacon, microwave ready meals, and cup noodles are normally low in nutrients and high in unhealthy chemicals.

As you can tell from the above list, a lot of unhealthy foods include foods that are processed/artificial. Try to stick with organic foods, moderate the amount of carbs you consume in your diet, and read ingredient lists. Checking the nutritional facts will help you see what contains sugar, wheat, and other ingredients that would impede on your weight loss journey.

Flavored Water/Drinks

Even though a lot of flavored drinks are proclaimed as great 'fitness drinks', many include considerable amounts of sugars or artificial sweeteners. If these flavored drinks contain unhealthy ingredients, it may be better to choose plain water instead.

Try MUFAs

In order to shed belly fat, it's good to eat some foods with monounsaturated fatty acids (MUFAs). Researchers found that when women were asked to switch to a 1,600-calorie, high-MUFA diet, they lost a third of their belly fat in a month. A serving of MUFAs like a handful of nuts, a tablespoon of olive oil, or a quarter of an avocado along with your daily foods would prove to burn belly fat.

Limit Your Alcohol Intake

Do not drink more than one drink a day and try to stay under 7 drinks a week. Drinking in moderation equates to 1 drink a day for a woman or 2 drinks a day for a man at maximum. But keep in mind, 3 beers a week can equate to an extra 1500 carb grams a year so try to reduce your intake as much as possible. Another thing to note, drinks don't "roll over". So if you're not drinking on weekdays but you're drinking over 7 drinks on a weekend, it's unfortunately not considered moderate drinking.

Don't Skip Out on This Miracle Mineral

Magnesium is more crucial for your body than you may have thought. The nutrient regulates more than 300 functions in the body and people who consume more of it tend to have lower blood sugar and insulin levels. So make it a habit of consuming magnesium-rich foods such as bananas, fish, dark green leafy vegetables, avocado, and soybeans at least twice a day for a healthier you.

How to Control Your Cravings with Other Food Replacements

Instead of creating a mindset of bidding farewell to your favorite pizzas, burgers, and other junk food, adopt an initial habit of eating healthy. The more you incline yourself to healthy food, the less appealing junk food will be. Like any other habit it takes time to adjust it into your daily regime, so be patient and stick to it. Adopt a healthy lifestyle and with time you will learn how to take control of your cravings.

Switch to Superfoods

Evidence shows superfoods have the capacity to help you with weight loss. Not only do they do this, but they are proven to build stronger bones, prevent chronic diseases, keep you quick on your toes, and improve your eyesight. Superfoods are termed as foods that supply your body with much-needed nutrients and include considerable health benefits to build a strong immune system. Here are some example superfoods that you can try:

Tomatoes: Full of potassium, fiber, vitamin C

Black beans: Contains heart-healthy fiber, antioxidants, and iron

Broccoli: Also has vitamin C, folic acid, reduces cancer risk.

Salmon: A rich source of selenium, vitamin B, and omega-3 fatty acids

Stay Hydrated

Water is one of the main secrets to healthy weight loss. It's shown that 60% of the time we feel hungry, we're actually thirsty but our mind translates it as hunger. Most people don't drink enough water on a daily basis. Drinking water will help you avoid eating as it will fill your stomach more, helping you eat less than your regular diet. To stay hydrated, try to consume around 2 liters of water a day (about 8 glasses). Drinking this much a day can help increase energy expenditure by over 96 calories a day.

Staying hydrated also plays an active role in boosting your metabolism, which helps cleanse waste from your body. A German study revealed that drinking a little more than a pint of cold water can enhance your metabolic rate by 30 percent for whole one hour. It is highly recommended to have a cup of lukewarm water after your meals to help remove unnecessary toxins from your body along with the oils you intake. This will help prevent fat from making itself at home in your body.

As a good practice, keep a bottle of water handy whenever you leave your house. At the same time, keep a pitcher full of water and cucumbers in your living room. It's refreshing and has a nice presence that makes it feel like you're treating yourself with each drink.Try to develop a habit of drinking water as much as you can before and during your meals to reduce your hunger and make you eat less than you normally would.

Replace Sugary Junk Foods with Dark Chocolate
Are you finding yourself guiltily eating Twix bars, Starbursts, or other junk foods from time to time? Try replacing these favorites with something containing a similar great taste that's healthier and tastier, like dark chocolate.

Why Dark Chocolate?
Sugary sweets make your body resistant to insulin which causes your body to produce more ghrelin, a hormone that increases your appetite. However, dark chocolate actually stops this insulin resistance and reduces ghrelin levels. People who eat dark chocolate tend to feel more full after each meal.

Furthermore, dark chocolate contains polyphenols and anandamides that positively impact your sense of well-being. It also contains chemicals that slow/stop the breakdown of anandamide so that the feeling of well-being stays longer.

Dark chocolate can be very good for reducing body fat if eaten moderately at about one ounce of dark chocolate 3 times a week. This also has to be paired with regular exercise and a healthy diet as losing weight still requires you to consume fewer calories than you burn.

Which Dark Chocolates Should You Eat or Avoid?

You'll still have to be careful about which dark chocolates are in fact good for you and which are not as much. Make sure to look at the below factors to make sure the dark chocolate you are consuming is indeed healthy:

1. Say no to anything labeled "made with chocolate" or "chocolate-coated", as it likely doesn't contain much cocoa butter, which is the ingredient you should look for with weight loss.

2. Say no to chocolates with more than 10 grams of sugar per ounce.

3. Say no to bars made with less than 70% cacao (the healthy ingredient in chocolate).

4. Try organic or milk-free dark chocolates rich in cocoa.

This dark chocolate replacement will help you indulge in your guilty pleasures, minus the guilt.

Beet Juice: The Best Substitute for Sugary Drinks

Beet juice contains low calories but substantial amounts of fiber that leave you feeling more full. Consuming beets and beet juice is one of the most effective, healthy, and natural weight-loss methods to help you reduce weight. While drinking beet juice, keep in mind that it isn't recommended to follow this diet for more than 10 days straight, and while you're consuming it you should remember to drink at least 2 liters of water a day.

Keep Fruits on You

Always try to keep a stash of fruits at work with you to meet your frequent cravings. It keeps you from going for junk food from time to time and also lets you adopt a healthy lifestyle. Make sure you fill up a daily bowl full of seasonal fruits including apples, oranges, papayas, pomegranates, etc. or keep them in your handbag each day.

Pizza Alternatives

If your idea of a relaxing weekend at home includes a couple of pizza slices and a glass of beer, you are definitely not alone. Although it's delicious, it's loaded with calories and fat. Therefore, we've compiled a few pizza alternatives to help satisfy your pizza cravings:

It might sound a bit unappealing at first, but try wrapping up a whole-wheat english muffin with your all-time favourite toppings. This is a "no cheat" pizza recipe and you'll get all the great tastes of pizza in one serving. This is among one of my favorite tricks to hinder the never ending cravings for the beloved pizza.

If a pizza alternative is not good enough for you, try whole-wheat pizza dough. It is a healthier substitute and you'll hardly notice the difference. Same goes for veggie crusts if you're trying to accomplish your weight loss goals and don't want to stop eating your favorite pizzas.

Want a better cheese substitute? Try soy cheese because it is lactose free and only contributes to 330 calories per serving, which is far lower than normal cheese.

How to Eat Healthy Using S.M.A.R.T. Goals

As previously mentioned, goal setting is crucial to losing weight. It's good practice to use S.M.A.R.T. goals for your healthy eating lifestyle. In order to do so, first check your weight. This will help you determine your nutrition goals. Next, use a calorie calculator tool to figure out how many calories your body needs so that you will have a daily goal in mind when reading food labels and keeping a food diary.

After these steps, write down your S.M.A.R.T. goals. Now that you've gotten a deeper understanding of what to eat, what not to eat, and what foods to consume to replace cravings, you should have no problem creating these objectives. However, in case you're having trouble, here are some examples that you can check out to give you ideas. You should write goals that really suit you, so make sure not to copy these examples exactly:

Water: Try drinking more water and less of other unhealthy drinks (like sodas and sweet juices). A sample goal would be: "I will only drink water and no other beverages for 1 month."

Portion Size: You can start reducing your meal portion sizes. A sample goal would be: "I will use an X sized plate for my meals and I will not get seconds for 1 month."

White Meat: Instead of eating dark meat or red meat, try eating white meats of chicken or turkey, which are lower in fat. Or, try eating pork tenderloin instead of high-fat meat. A sample would be: "I will eat white meat instead of dark meat or red meat for 1 month."

Vegetables: Vegetables need to be incorporated in your meals. A sample goal would be: "I will eat at least 1 cup of vegetables for lunch and 1 cup of vegetables for dinner every day for 1 month."

Daily Life Tips

We've covered what to eat for a healthy lifestyle. As you know from the weight loss equation, you have to not only consume less calories but burn more calories as well. In order to get lasting results, you must consistently exercise and stay committed

Rise Early

According to various studies, people who exercise in the morning are more likely to stick to their workouts than those who exercise later in the day. When you postpone your workouts until the evening, it is common that you'll deplete your energy by that time and will be lazier about your workout.

When you're trying to wake up early for workouts, it's common to find yourself unable to rise for the occasion even when setting an alarm. In order to avoid this situation, try to keep your alarm clock far away from your bed, so you can't avoid getting out of bed to turn it off. Once you are out of your bed, it is not that difficult to go for a workout. It might be hard to stay consistent with this, but opting for a workout first thing in the morning would induce a positive energy that normally lasts the whole of your day. Workouts, if left for the later half of the day, are not as effective when you're more easily occupied with distractions.

Be Patient

It's important to be patient after setting your fitness goals. Changes to your body are not seen instantly as it takes a few months after consistent work. When you stay patient and start seeing results, you're going to want to continue working out out of your own interest.

Find Your Workout of Choice

Choose only the type of workouts that would work for you. Some people are more into dance or sports, while others prefer exercising at the gym. If you are not comfortable with one particular type of workout, try switching to a different one. Go for something that allows you to enjoy yourself while relieving stress.

Choose A Workout Place of Convenience
You're more likely to exercise if you choose a place that's convenient to visit for your workouts. Some may feel comfortable working out at home, some at the gym, and others may find a nearby park to be their place of convenience. If you decide to go to a place that is far away from your dwelling, then likelihood of going will decrease immensely.

Emphasize on Quality instead of Quantity
It's shown that some of the best workouts are actually 20 minutes or less. Focus on quality instead of quantity. We tend to think that the longer our workout, the more calories burned. For example, it's assumed that a 60 minute run is better than a 20 minute workout which is not always the case. Try workouts with multidimensional movement and high intensity exercise so you can get the most out of less time. We'll go over some of these exercises below.

Get Techy
If you are tech savvy, you should especially try fitness apps and online health trackers that notify you about the ins and outs of calories. This in turn would help you to effectively plan your goals. There are wearable pedometers as well that can help you stay on track with your routines. With the help of these tools you will not only be able to keep track of daily number of calories burned but you'll continuously challenge yourself to new personal bests every day.

Bike or Run At a Sweat-Inducing Pace
If you are fond of biking or running, make sure you accelerate at a pace that makes it hard to talk for two minutes, then slow down for a minute, and repeat until you're done - similar to resistance training. Make sure whatever activities you are going to perform should not involve lengthy breaks in between. Instead, you should make sure you're releasing sweat from your body with your workouts..

Counter Depression/Sadness with Exercise

Many who become depressed or sad tend to eat more and exercise less. Rather than fall into bad habits, use exercise to counter depression. By forcing yourself to move physically, you're keeping your mind on other more productive things so you'll be less likely to succumb to your negative feelings. Also, when you exercise your body releases endorphins, which are chemicals that react with the brain to reduce your perception of pain. This then triggers a positive feeling and outlook on life, which helps combat your sadness.

Another way of combating a habit of consuming excessive foods when depressed is keeping around a bowl of fruits or healthy snacks and grabbing it whenever your hunger hits. We're constantly tempted by junk food, but what it comes down to is self control. Because we're generally a lazy species, we're more likely to eat whatever's in front of us - so stock up on your fruits and salads!

Treat Yourself

Treat yourself once in a while after a great workout. Let yourself have your favorite guilty pleasure foods at least once a week so you don't drive yourself crazy trying to replace junk foods for healthy foods. And try to associate positive experiences with your exercises - for example, play your favorite playlist of songs that you'll only listen to while you run or jog. Or, turn on your favorite TV show that you'll only play while running on your treadmill. When you associate positivity to your workouts, you're more likely going to look forward to your daily exercises and look at them as less of a burden.

Take Walks Between Work and Before Meals

It's not news that walking is great for your health. If you're stuck at a desk and sitting on a chair all day, 5-10 minutes of walking every 2-3 hours can do wonders for you. I like to take this walk between work and before lunch and dinner. Taking walks during your lunch break can dramatically improve your mood for the rest of the day and allow you to handle stress better.

Do Your Chores Once a Week

According to studies a 150-pound person will burn about four calories per minute spent cleaning. One hour of cleaning, including acts of bending over to pick things up and reaching into cabinets, burns an average of 238 calories. Mopping can burn about 119 calories per half hour. And washing the dishes can burn about 85 calories per half an hour. Try regularly participating in your weekly errands like cleaning, laundry, dishes, etc. I find myself always doing chores as it keeps my house clean and makes me feel good knowing I'm burning calories at the same time! Productivity feels good.

Don't Give Into Fake Trainers

Losing weight is not an overnight task; it involves a lot of commitment, hard work, and for many, a complete lifestyle makeover. So if anyone is telling you that you can lose 10 pounds in 10 days, the trainer is most likely trying to bait you into joining his or her program - don't trust the lies! Even if it might be partially true the weight you lose most likely won't last. There is no use in losing weight that will only be regained as it will demotivate you and push you into the wrong mentality.

Get a Fitness Trainer

Though you'll come across those BS trainers, don't give up on the idea completely. Trainers can be of great help if you have the money for it. No matter what, if you're a newcomer to the fitness scene or if you just need a little motivation and guidance, a personal trainer can guide you through all aspects of setting feasible goals, creating a plan, and forcing you to execute to make them happen. Be picky when choosing a trainer. If your first choice of a fitness trainer doesn't suit you, keep looking and don't settle for less.

Practically speaking, however, many of us can't afford a good fitness trainer to help us achieve our weight loss goals. But this does not mean that you are short of options; there are many ways to self train..

Switch to Sound Sleep

Make sure to get 7-9 hours of sleep a day. When you're not getting enough sleep, your brain is constantly looking for things that feel good to appease the tiredness. Studies have found that lack of sleep is associated with cravings for high carb snacks, bigger portions for meals, and more frequent lattes that all lead to weight gain. This happens because lack of sleep causes your body to make more ghrelin (which signals your brain to eat) and also reduces leptin levels (the hormone that tells your brain to stop eating).

Not only does sleep affect your hunger levels, it also affects your metabolism. Little sleep also causes you to release cortisol which signals your body to conserve energy to fuel your awake time - AKA you're likely to hang onto fat. When sleep deprived, your body will also be 30% less capable of processing insulin, which is needed to change starches, sugar into energy. Your body then isn't able to process fat from the bloodstream and the fat ends up being stored.

Exercises Routines

I've gathered some great exercises I personally use, which will not only help you in your weight loss journey but will also help you feel healthier and build confidence. These exercises are cost effective weight loss options that don't even require the use of fitness equipment.

Planking

To plank, get into pushup position, bend your elbows 90 degrees, and rest your weight on your forearms. This is an elementary move that you can follow to keep yourself fit and give you rock hard abs.

This exercise works the abdominal muscles and lower back.

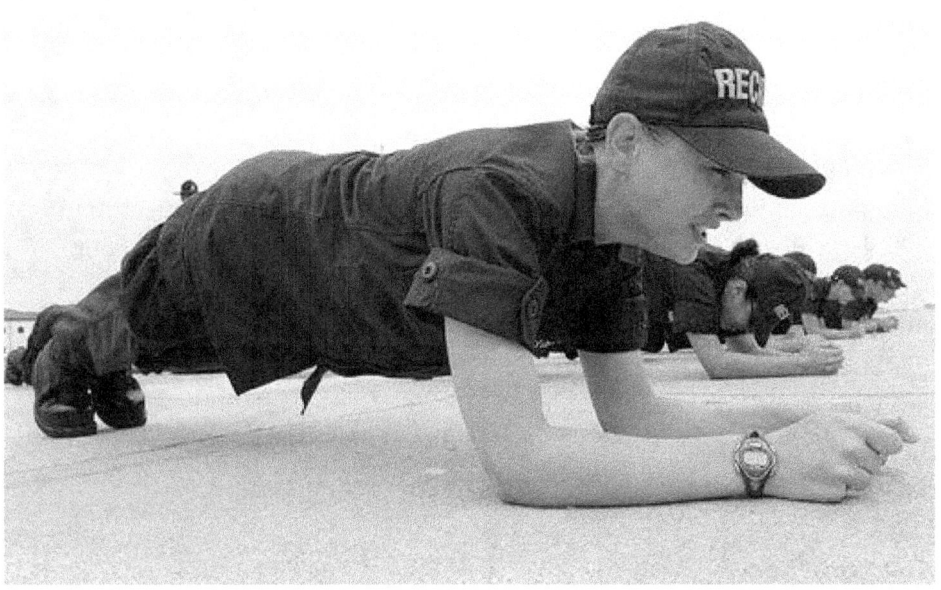

Jumping Jacks

Jumping jacks are among one of the most effective cardio moves that you can go for, and it especially works the shoulders, abs, and leg muscles. Doing this exercise on a daily basis will help you burn off excessive fat from your entire body.

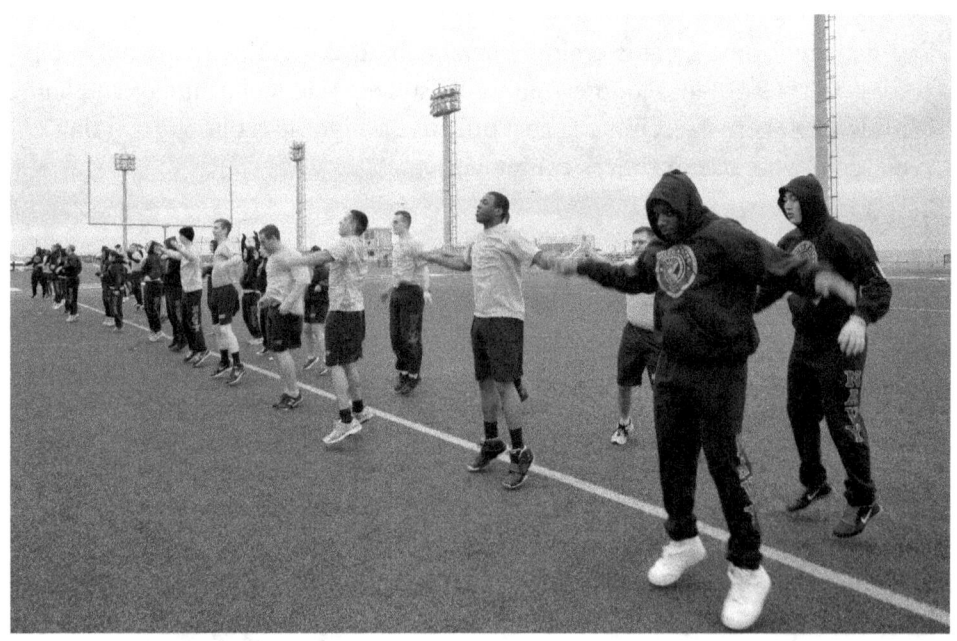

Skipping/Jump Roping

Skipping and jump roping are good cardio exercises that can burn around 300-400 calories in 45 minutes depending upon your body weight. Jump roping will burn off around 720 calories in an hour at 120-140 turns per minute, about the same as running close six miles. It is also proven that 10 minutes of skipping can have health benefits equivalent to 30 minutes of running.

Skipping and jump roping work the muscles in the calves.

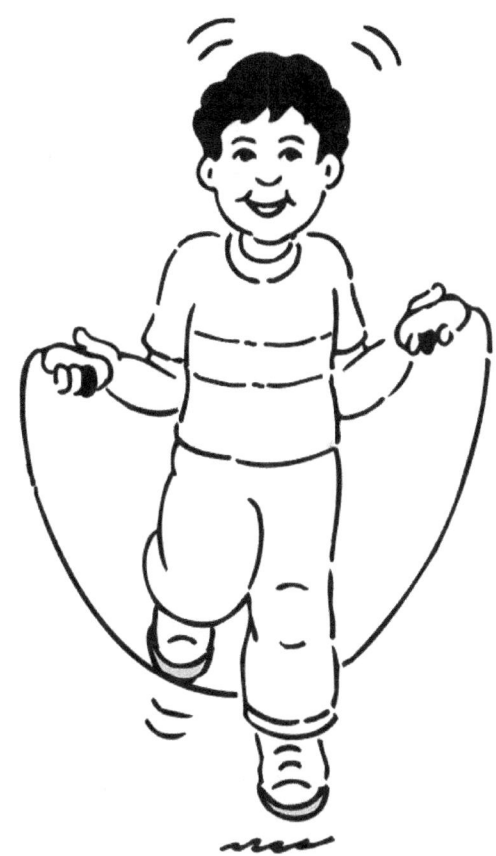

Glute Bridges

With glute bridges, lay on your back with your legs bent, feet on the ground, and hands to your sides. Dig your heels into the ground and lift your pelvis up. Make sure your knees, pelvis, and shoulders are aligned in a straight line. Hold this bridge, and lift your right knee toward your chest until your thigh makes a 90 degree angle with your stomach. Return the heel and lift the left knee. Do 2 sets of 6 reps of this. This exercise works the glutes, hamstrings, and spinal muscles in the lower back.

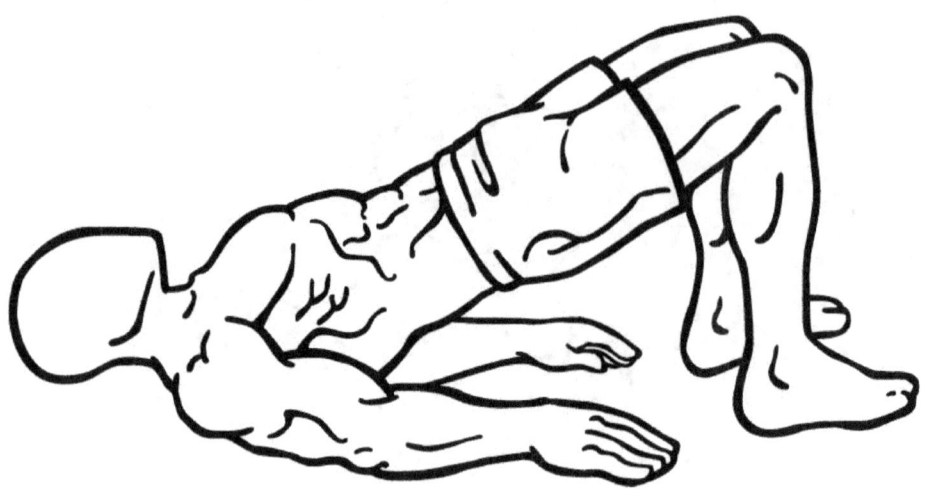

Butt Kicks

Butt kicks are cardiovascular exercises that aim to work on your hamstrings and glutes. The difference between butt kicks and jogging is that in butt kicks, you try to kick up to the glutes alternatively with each leg. The knees should not come in front of the body, and the arms should swing with the opposite leg at 90 degrees, alternately. There should not be any side to side movement. You can perform this exercise while jogging in place or jogging over a distance.

Conclusion

A few adjustments to your eating habits and exercise regimen can do wonders for your body. This guide should push you towards become a better version of yourself. It's not just about shedding a few pounds. It's about making sure you're living a healthy lifestyle so you can feel good about yourself and ultimately live a longer life. Your body's a temple. You have to treat it with respect!

My whole life has changed for the better after following these steps. It was a challenging journey, no doubt about it. It took me so long to realize that this was something I truly needed to change about myself and had to put in full effort for. The hardest part was committing. The whole experience is a journey and requires months of consistency, but it is truly rewarding. And when you commit, the exercise routines and diet regimen will become a part of your life that you'll voluntarily want. So start changing your life today and take action! Create your S.M.A.R.T. goals and commit to a better 'you'.

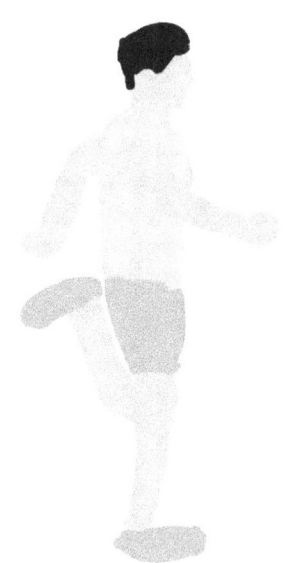

Intense Cardio

Intense 45-minute cardio sessions if done effectively a few times a week, can help in boosting your body's metabolism. Research shows that an intense cardio session can burn an additional 190 calories. Some intense cardio workouts to try include indoor cycling or treadmill running.

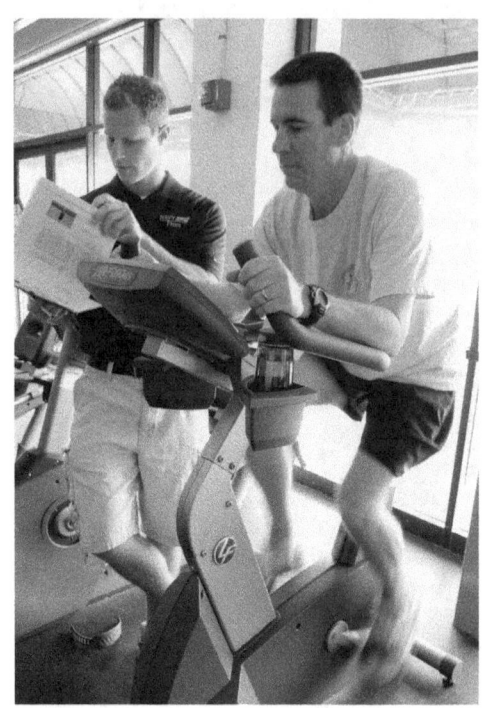

Yoga

Yoga is an ancient spiritual science developed thousands of years ago, and the practice can actually mean many different things. It is often seen as a type of light physical activity but in reality it's a blend of physical, mental and spiritual exercises which if performed in sync may bring many positive benefits.

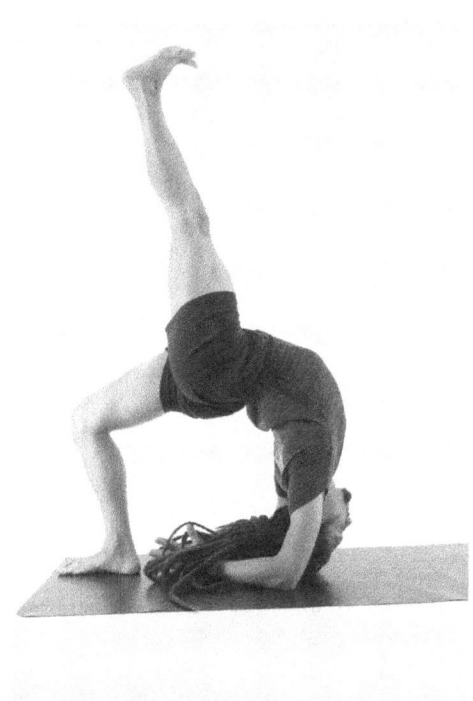

Yoga is a great exercise for losing weight. There are different types of yoga including Ashtanga, Vinyasa or Power Yoga which involve more physical exercise that will help you burn calories, tone your body, and strengthen your muscles. Yoga thickens the layers of the cerebral cortex (part of the brain which is associated with higher learning) and increases neuroplasticity. This helps us transform our way of living to help us deal with day to day things.

Some may ask if yoga is intense enough to really shed pounds. I find the most important benefit of yoga in terms of weight loss is its ability to help you control your appetite. Not only does it burn calories, but it also helps you learn "mindfulness", which is a state of equilibrium between your body and mind that will encourage you to opt for healthy food choices. You become more in tune with your body as yoga develops a firm mind-body connection that makes you more aware of your eating habits. Mindfulness will also result in actual implementation of healthy practices.

Stress and worry sometimes consume your mind, which in turn make us more psychologically prone to consume more than our normal diet. Yoga serves as a perfect stress buster which keeps you away from unnecessary day-to-day anxiety.

S.M.A.R.T. Fitness Goals

Learning more about exercise routines and regular daily tips, it's important to create S.M.A.R.T. goals again to keep yourself on track with your workouts. Below are some example goals, and again, make sure your goals are tailored to yourself.

Morning run: "I will wake up 30 minutes earlier than normal and run for 20 minutes on the treadmill before work."

Walking: "I will walk 15 minutes a day during my lunch breaks at work."

General exercise goal: "I will exercise for 30 minutes a day."

Specific exercise goal: "I will do 2 sets of 6 reps of glute bridges and 20 minutes of butt kicks per day."

How to Stay Motivated

Getting fit and staying fit are two different stories. With the previously explained tips and tricks you'll understand the steps to take to reduce weight in a healthy manner. But it's much easier to get fit and a lot harder to stay fit, which requires determination, persistence, and commitment.

In this last section, I want to make sure you stay motivated with everything you're doing. You HAVE to keep practicing a healthier lifestyle in order to maintain results. This lifestyle makeover may initially feel forced and difficult. But the thing with consistency is you'll start developing a normal inclination to your routine and will want to pursue your routines willingly. One of my friends used to always eat junk food and exercise very infrequently. After implementing some of these practices he started WILLINGLY avoiding pizzas and fast food. The foods didn't taste the same to him anymore - he started feeling a bit disgusted by them. He would only drink around 3 drinks a week (as opposed to his regular binge drinking practices). And he would hit the gym every day. It became a lifestyle makeover that was not forced, but wanted. You can do the same, if you keep up with these practices.

Use Mantras for Motivation
Fitness mantras work quite well. Start telling yourself things like "consistency is key" or "paralyze resistance with persistence" and repeating S.M.A.R.T. goals to yourself. Remember your overall goals with your weight loss journey, which may include a healthier lifestyle and toned body. When you continue ingraining your purpose in your head you'll start thinking smarter about each food and exercise choice you make. You'll find motivation from these sayings. Rather than thinking about foods you can't resist, start thinking about why you started your weight loss journey in the first place. Reminding yourself of why you started your journey will keep you fighting for your goals.

Place These Mantras Around Your House

After setting your mantras, start putting up reminders wherever you can - whether it be via posters, notes on the fridge, or writings in your notebook. Make sure these reminders and frequently visited. Through these means, constantly tell yourself you're on a journey and remember the end goal. Your S.M.A.R.T. goals should be placed around the house and on mobile apps as well (like Google Keep) so you'll constantly see them.

Find Your Best Fitness Partners

Try to surround yourself with people who care about health and fitness and are on a similar path as you. They will serve as inspiration to meet your milestones. Working out with these people helps a lot, as through each other's support, you'll keep track of each other as to not skip a day at the gym or break your cycle of healthy eating.

www.ingramcontent.com/pod-product-compliance
Lightning Source LLC
Chambersburg PA
CBHW072019280526
45788CB00007B/2618